Table of Contents

What are the symptoms of Graves' disease?

Graves' disease and hyperthyroidism share many of the same symptoms.

These symptoms can include:

- rapid heart rate (tachycardia)
- hand tremors
- heat sensitivity or intolerance
- weight loss
- sleep problems, including difficulty sleeping and fatigue
- nervousness and irritability
- muscle weakness
- goiter (swelling in your thyroid gland)
- fre uent formed bowel movements
- irregular periods

- difficulty becoming pregnant

- Graves' dermopathy

Some people with Graves' disease will experience Graves' dermopathy.

With this condition, you'll notice reddened, thickened skin around your shins or on the tops of your feet. While Graves' dermopathy is often mild, it can potentially cause some pain and discomfort.

Graves' opthalmopathy

Graves' disease can also cause Graves' ophthalmopathy (GO).

This condition develops when your immune system begins to attack eye tissue and muscle, leaving your eye sockets swollen and inflamed. This inflammation can cause your eyelids to retract, which makes your eyes seem enlarged and bulging.

You might also notice:

- blurred or double vision
- irritated or dry eyes
- sensitivity to light
- pain or a sense of pressure in your eyes

The National Institute of Diabetes and Digestive and Kidney Diseases (NIDDK) estimates that about 30 percent of people who develop Graves' disease will get a mild case of GO. Up to 5 percent will have more severe symptoms.

Mild cases of GO might improve on their own. Yet since rare complications can include vision loss, it's best to mention any eye symptoms you experience to your care team, even mild ones. Be sure to follow any

recommended treatment guidelines.

5

What causes Graves' disease?

Your immune system usually produces proteins known as antibodies in order to fight against foreign invaders like viruses and bacteria.

If you have an autoimmune disease like Graves' disease, though, your immune system begins to fight against healthy tissues and cells in your body.

With Graves' disease, instead of producing antibodies to target a specific invader, your immune system mistakenly produces thyroid-stimulating immunoglobulins. These antibodies then target your own healthy thyroid cells.

Scientists know that people can inherit the ability to make antibodies against their own healthy cells. But they have yet to find a clear cause of Graves' disease or determine who will develop it.

Experts believe it's possible that your genes and a virus or other external trigger both play a part in its development.

Who is at risk of Graves' disease?

A few different factors may affect your chance of developing Graves' disease:

- genetics (family history of the condition)
- stress
- age
- gender

The disease typically develops in people younger than 40. Your risk also increases significantly if any family members have Graves' disease. The NIDDK says that women develop it 7 to 8 times more fre uently than men.

Your risk also increases if you have another autoimmune disease. Examples include:

- rheumatoid arthritis
- type 1 diabetes
- Crohn's disease

How is Graves' disease diagnosed?

Your doctor may re uest laboratory tests if they think you might have Graves' disease. If anyone in your family has had Graves' disease, your doctor may be able to narrow down the diagnosis based on your medical history and a physical examination.

They'll still need to confirm the diagnosis through thyroid blood tests. A doctor who specializes in diseases related to hormones, known as an endocrinologist, may handle your tests and diagnosis.

Your doctor may also re uest some of the following tests:

- blood test
- thyroid ultrasound
- radioactive iodine uptake test

- thyroid-stimulating hormone test

- thyroid-stimulating immunoglobulin test

The combined results of these may help your doctor learn if you have Graves' disease or another type of thyroid disorder.

How is Graves' disease treated?

Three treatment options are available for people with Graves' disease:

- antithyroid drugs
- radioactive iodine therapy
- thyroid surgery

Your care team may suggest using one or more of these options to treat the condition.

Antithyroid drugs

Your doctor may prescribe antithyroid drugs, including propylthiouracil and methimazole, or beta-blockers.

Beta-blockers don't treat the condition itself, but they can help lower the effects of your symptoms until other treatments begin to work.

Radioactive iodine therapy

Radioactive iodine therapy is one of the most common treatments for Graves' disease. This treatment requires you to take doses of radioactive iodine-131.

This usually re uires you to swallow small amounts in pill form. Your doctor will explain any important precautions for you to take with this therapy.

Thyroid surgery

Although thyroid surgery is an option, your doctor may not suggest it right away. They may recommend surgery if previous treatments haven't worked or if they suspect you could have thyroid cancer, though thyroid cancer is rare with Graves' disease.

They might also recommend thyroid surgery if you're pregnant and can't take antithyroid drugs. In this case, they'll wait to do the surgery until your second trimester because of the risk of miscarriage.

If surgery is necessary, your doctor will remove your entire thyroid gland, a procedure known as a total thyroidectomy. The goal of this surgery is to eliminate the risk of hyperthyroidism returning. Total thyroidectomy is the standard of care for people with Graves' disease.

After surgery, you'll need thyroid hormone replacement therapy on an ongoing basis.

How Graves' Disease Develops

Normally, thyroid-stimulating hormone (TSH) is released by the pituitary gland in the brain and usually determines how much hormones the thyroid produces. But people with Graves' disease experience a break in normal communication between the pituitary glad and thyroid gland, resulting in abnormal antibodies being released that mimic TSH and therefore cause too much thyroid hormone to be circulated into the bloodstream.

These antibodies are called thyroid stimulating immunoglobulin (TSI) and thyrotropin receptor antibody (TRAb). TSI cells have a similar effect to TSH, which we need in ade uate amounts to help the thyroid function normally. But TSI antibodies cause the thyroid gland to produce excess thyroid hormones above and beyond what is necessary and healthy.

Since the thyroid mistakes these antibodies for TSH, they can override normal signals sent from the pituitary gland and therefore cause hyperthyroidism. As TSI and TRAb levels rise, inflammation increases, which indicates that the immune system is working on overdrive and accidentally attacking the body's own healthy tissue. A harmful cycle can develop in people with Graves' disease because the more active the immune system becomes, the more bodily tissue is damaged and then more activated T-cells and auto-antibodies are released.

We produce several different kinds of thyroid hormones normally, including the types called T3 and T4. Compared to healthy people without autoimmune or thyroid disorders, on a blood test people with

Graves' disease show abnormally high levels of T3 and T4, low TSH, and a high presence of TSI antibodies.

Some of the most noticeable effects of Graves' disease are changes in someone's weight, mood and appearance. That's because hormones secreted by the thyroid gland control your metabolism — meaning your body's ability to use nutrients and calories from the food you eat in order to have enough energy. You've likely heard and noticed that genetics play a big part in determining someone's body weight. That's because thyroid gland activity is somewhat hereditary — therefore so is the rate of someone's metabolism. The metabolic rate is determined by the amount of available circulating thyroid hormones. So when the thyroid gland secretes an overabundance of these hormones, the metabolism can shoot up and cause weight loss, anxiousness and irritability.

A link also has been identified between Graves' disease and another thyroid disorder known as Hashimoto's thyroiditis. Hashimoto's is the most common cause of hypothyroidism and, like Graves' disease, it's also an autoimmune disorder. Hashimoto's can sometimes develop after taking antithyroid medication as a treatment for Graves' disease as the medication causes the thyroid to slow production of thyroid hormones and move towards hypothyroidism.

Graves' Disease: 7 Ways to Help Manage Hyperthyroid Symptoms

Manage Stress Levels

Several studies, involving both humans and animals, show that stress can ignite autoimmune reactions and worsen inflammation. That's probably why such a high percentage of Graves' disease patients report having experienced trauma or chronic stress before developing the disease. Research demonstrates that stress causes both physical and psychological changes that impact how the immune system works, causing a downstream of neuro-endocrine alterations that can wind up leading to autoimmune disorders and tissue damage.

Stress can raise levels of cortisol and adrenaline, which disturb neurotransmitter function and worsen symptoms of thyroid disease. To keep stress from aggravating Graves' disease, build stress-reducing practices into your day, including natural stress relievers such as: exercise, meditation, prayer, spending time in nature, using essential oils, massage therapy, acupuncture or volunteering for a good cause.

Eat an Anti-inflammatory Diet

Reducing inflammation through a healthy diet is one of the best ways to enhance immune function, create a healthy gut environment and manage your autoimmune symptoms. Inflammation can partially be traced to an unhealthy gut "microbiota" that is caused by nutrient deficiencies, food allergies or sensitivities, which all raise autoimmune activity.

Some of the ways that your diet might trigger autoimmune reactions include eating common allergens like gluten and dairy products, which the immune system can actually register as a threat when they aren't digested properly. Allergens can contribute to leaky gut syndrome, in which small particles leak out into the bloodstream through tiny openings in the gut lining, triggering autoimmunity.

A well-rounded diet that's filled with anti-inflammatory foods and free from toxin overload helps resolve bacterial imbalances in the gut that make symptoms worse.

Focus on limiting or avoiding foods capable of aggravating autoimmune disorders, including:

- conventional dairy products
- gluten

- artificial flavorings or dyes

- added sugar

GMO ingredients (common in almost all packaged foods which contain preservatives, high fructose corn syrup and other chemical ingredients)

It's also important to avoid foods that are high in iodine as it increases levels of thyroid hormone. These include foods such as iodized salt, egg yolks and seaweed. For this same reason, avoid certain herbs and plants, including bladderwrack (a sea plant). Some herbs also have thyroid-stimulating properties, such as ashwaganda. Speak with your natural health care practitioner or herbalist before taking herbal supplements.

Foods that can help control Graves' disease symptoms include:

- fresh vegetables/green juices: these provide vital nutrients and fight inflammation
- fresh fruit: a great source of antioxidants and electrolytes, but avoid processed fruit juices
- anti-inflammatory herbs: basil, rosemary, parsley and oregano are all anti-inflammatory
- spices like tumeric, garlic and ginger: known to help boost immune system function
- bone broth: helps heal the gut and improve detoxification
- probiotics: balance bacteria within the digestive tract and fight leaky gut syndrome
- healthy fats including omega-3s: lower inflammation and helps with neurotransmitter functions

Get Some Exercise

Exercise is a great way to help control stress and lower inflammation, as long as it's enjoyable and doesn't involve overtraining, which may make you even more irritable. Do some sort of exercise daily that makes you feel happier, less anxious and hopefully helps you sleep. Soothing exercises that can work well include dancing, yoga, cycling or swimming. Listening to music while exercising is another great way to "get into the zone" and feel more relaxed afterward.

Another reason to eat a nutrient-rich diet and to exercise is to help protect your bones, since having a thyroid disorder already interferes with your ability to maintain bone strength. Having very high levels of thyroid hormone interferes with your body's normal ability to incorporate calcium or other minerals into your bones. This means you need to do whatever you can to lower bone loss in other ways. Strength training, including doing bodyweight exercises at home, helps keep bones strong as you age.

Quit Smoking

Cigarette smoking and exposure to tobacco and other recreational drugs has been found to be a potential trigger for autoimmune disorders, including Graves' disease. It's not exactly clear how cigarettes might make Graves' disease worse, but it's very likely that the high amount of toxins present in cigarettes (and other drugs) raises inflammation, damages healthy cells and tissue, and therefore activates the immune system to release more T-fighter cells.

Lower Exposure to Environmental Toxins

Most of us come into contact with various chemical or environmental toxins multiple times every single day. There are over 80,000 chemicals and toxins used legally every single year in the U.S. in common household or beauty products, chemically-sprayed crops, prescription medications, birth control pills, and antibiotics. These can all wind up accumulating in the water supply and elsewhere, making their way into our homes and bodies.

I recommend buying organic produce as much as possible, using natural household products (including essential oils), avoiding unnecessary medications however you can, and drinking high- uality water that's been filtered to eliminate chlorine and fluoride.

Treat Sensitivity of the Eyes and Skin

If you develop Graves' complications in the eyes or on the skin, there are some simple remedies you can try at home to ease inflammation and pain. One particular complication that can occur with this disease is Graves' ophthalmopathy, also known as Graves' orbitopathy, which causes the eyes to bulge and can cause vision problems. It can also cause dry, puffy eyes, sometimes with a sensation of grittiness. Try using a cool compress pressed against your eyes to keep them moisturized, as well as applying lubricating eyes drops. Also, always wear sunglasses when outdoors, since sensitive eyes are more prone to damage from ultraviolet rays. If your eyes become puffy overnight, try raising your head while you're sleeping to keep blood and fluid from building up around your face.

If Graves' affects your skin, you can use soothing essential oils combined with coconut oil to fight itchiness, swelling and reddening. Essential oils that are gentle and anti-inflammatory include lavender, frankincense, rose and tea tree oil.

Talk to Your Doctor About Potential Graves' Disease Complications

There are certain complications that develop when Graves' disease is untreated. This is especially true if you're pregnant, have other forms of inflammatory diseases or if you suffer from another autoimmune disorder.

If you're pregnant, it's important to get Graves' under control since it raises the risk for miscarriage, preterm birth, fetal thyroid dysfunction, poor fetal growth, maternal heart failure and preeclampsia (high blood pressure). If you have a history of heart disease or complications, Graves' disease can lead to heart rhythm disorders, changes in the structure and function of the heart muscles, and even lead to possible heart failure in some rare cases. Also, because the high thyroid hormone levels can impact bone density, it's important to discuss the risk of osteoporosis (weak, brittle bones) with your doctor as well.

While there's plenty you can do on your own to lower Graves' disease risks and symptoms, always make sure to get professional help if you notice symptoms worsening suddenly or you're under a lot of stress/anxiety, which can trigger a relapse. Luckily, if it's treated, and at least mostly resolved, Graves' disease isn't likely to cause permanent damage or lead to other disorders.

The Best Diet for People with Graves' Disease

The foods you eat can't cure you of Graves' disease, but they can provide antioxidants and nutrients that may help alleviate symptoms or reduce flares.

Graves' disease causes the thyroid gland to produce too much thyroid hormone, which can result in hyperthyroidism. Certain symptoms associated with hyperthyroidism include:

- extreme weight loss, despite eating normally
- brittle bones and osteoporosis

Diet plays a big factor in managing Graves' disease. Some foods may exacerbate Graves' disease symptoms. Food sensitivities or allergies may negatively impact the immune system, causing disease flares in some people. For this reason, it's important to try to identify the foods you might be allergic to. Avoiding these foods may lessen symptoms.

Foods to avoid

Talk to your doctor or to a dietitian to help determine which foods you should avoid. You might also keep a food diary to track which foods aggravate your symptoms and which foods don't. Some types of food to consider eliminating include:

Gluten

There is a higher incidence of Celiac disease in people who have thyroid disease than there is in the general population. This may be due, in part, to a genetic link. Foods containing gluten may make treatment more difficult for people with autoimmune thyroid diseases, including Graves' disease. Many foods and drinks contain gluten. It's important to read labels and to look for gluten-containing ingredients. These include:

- wheat and wheat products
- rye
- barley
- malt
- triticale
- brewer's yeast
- grains of all kinds such as spelt, kamut, farro, and durum

Dietary iodine

There is some that excessive iodine intake might trigger hyperthyroidism in older adults or people who have a preexisting thyroid disease. Iodine is a micronutrient that is necessary for good health, so taking in the right amount is important. Discuss how much iodine you need with your doctor.

Iodine-fortified foods include:

- salt
- bread
- dairy products, such as milk, cheese, and yogurt

Foods which are naturally high in iodine include:
- seafood, especially white fish, such as haddock, and cod seaweed, and other sea vegetables, such as kelp

Avoiding meat and other animal products

One study found evidence that vegetarians had lower rates of hyperthyroidism than those who followed a non-vegetarian diet. The study found the greatest benefit in people who avoided all animal products, including meat, chicken, pork, and fish.

Foods to eat

Foods containing specific nutrients can help reduce some of the symptoms associated with Graves' disease. These include:

Calcium-rich foods

Hyperthyroidism can make it difficult for your body to absorb calcium. This can cause brittle bones and osteoporosis. Eating a diet high in calcium may help, although some dairy products are fortified with iodine and may not be as beneficial for you as others.

Since you need some iodine in your diet, it's important to talk to your doctor or dietitian about which dairy products you should eat, and which you should avoid. Other types of food that contain calcium include:

- broccoli
- almonds
- kale
- sardines
- okra

Foods high in vitamin D

Vitamin D helps your body absorb calcium from food more readily. Most vitamin D is made in the skin through the absorption of sunlight. Dietary sources include:

- sardines

- cod liver oil

- salmon

- tuna

- mushrooms

Foods high in magnesium

If your body doesn't have enough magnesium, it can affect its ability to absorb calcium. A magnesium deficiency may also worsen symptoms associated with Graves' disease. Foods high in this mineral include:

- avocados

- dark chocolate

- almonds

- brazil nuts

- cashews

- legumes

- pumpkin seeds

Foods containing selenium

A deficiency in selenium is associated with thyroid eye disease in people with Graves' disease. This can cause bulging eyeballs and double vision. Selenium is an antioxidant and a mineral. It can be found in:

- mushrooms
- brown rice
- brazil nuts
- sunflower seeds
- sardines

1. Creamy Cashew Matcha Dressing

Ingredients

1/2 cup soaked raw organic cashews, rinsed and drained*

2 tablespoons + 1 teaspoon lemon juice

1/2 cup + 2 tablespoons filtered water

1 teaspoon matcha powder

1 scoop collagen peptides

1/4 teaspoon ground ginger

Himalayan sea salt, to taste

Instructions

Place cashews in a bowl and cover with water.

Soak cashews at least 30 minutes or overnight.

When ready to blend, place all ingredients in a high powered blender or Vitamix and blend until smooth and creamy.

Transfer to a glass mason jar or glass container and drizzle on your favorite salad or use as a topping or marinade for chicken, shrimp, fish or tofu.

2. Easy Turmeric Chia Pudding

Ingredients

1 cup full-fat coconut milk or almond milk yogurt

1 scoop collagen peptides (optional)

2 tablespoons black or white chia seeds

dash of cinnamon

1 scoop Further Food Superfood Turmeric

Optional toppings: unsweetened flaked coconut, goji berries, cacao nibs, sliced banana, slivered raw almonds, or berries (optional)

Instructions

Mix all ingredients in a small bowl or mini mason jar.

Let sit in the refrigerator for 1 hour or more until the chia seeds expand into a "gel."

Top with unsweetened flaked coconut, goji berries, cacao nibs, sliced banana, slivered raw almonds, or berries (optional). Enjoy!

3. Creamy Butternut S uash Soup

Ingredients

2 tablespoons olive oil for roasting S uash

1 butternut s uash, 2-3 pounds or 1 package of pre-cut s uash

2 tablespoons olive oil

2 cloves garlic, chopped

2 cups of canned full-fat coconut milk

1 cup chicken stock (or vegetable stock for vegan option) or bone broth

2 teaspoons Superfood Turmeric

Himalayan sea salt and pepper to taste

Optional toppings: parsley, sage, cilantro, raw unshelled pumpkin seeds

Optional: 4 scoops Collagen Peptides

Instructions

Preheat the oven to 400F.

Peel & cube the squash. Coat with 2 Tablespoons of oil & season with salt. Place on a parchment covered baking sheet & roast for 45 minutes, turning the s uash at least once during roasting, so they'll be well caramelized.

Once finished, remove squash from the oven & set aside.

In a cast iron pot, add 2 Tablespoons of olive oil & sauté the garlic until fragrant.

Add the roasted s uash, coconut milk & stock or bone broth. Add collagen peptides if desired. With an immersion blender, blend until smooth.

Add in the turmeric powder & season with salt to taste.

Serve in bowls & top a drizzle of coconut milk or coconut cream, fresh herbs and pumpkin seeds.

Quick & Easy Version: Use 1 package of frozen butternut s uash, thawed. Add to a high-speed Vitamix or blender with all other ingredients and blend on high until smooth. Heat and serve warm when ready to eat. Add fresh herbs and pumpkin seeds as a garnish.

4. **Superfood Cashew**

Ingredients

1 large organic carrot, or about 1-2 cups of baby carrots

1 cup of organic raw cashews, pre-soaked in warm water before blending

2 tablespoons nutritional yeast

1 scoop Further Food Daily Turmeric Tonic

1 scoop FurtherFood Collagen Peptides

1/4 cup filtered water

Instructions

Soak nuts in lukewarm water for about 1 hour and drain before blending all ingredients.

Serve immediately or store in the refrigerator for up to one week.

5. Acorn S uash Shepherd's Pie

Ingredients

1 acorn s uash

¼ cup water

1 zucchini, diced

½ cup onion, minced

3 garlic cloves, minced

1 tbsp coconut oil

1 lb ground grass-fed beef or bison

Salt and pepper to taste

½ tsp ground thyme

½ tsp ground sage

2 cups bone broth

2 cups spinach

¼ cup coconut cream

Instructions

Preheat oven to 400 degrees F. Cut s uash in half and place in baking dish, flesh side down. Add ¼ cup water to bottom of the pan to help steam s uash as it cooks. Cook s uash in oven for about 45 minutes or until tender and cooked through.

Dice onion, garlic, and zucchini. Preheat large skillet on stovetop over medium-high heat. Add coconut oil and onion and garlic. Allow to cook until tender and translucent. Add meat to pan and sprinkle with salt, pepper, sage, and thyme. Cook meat until browned.

Once meat has browned, add zucchini, spinach, and bone broth to pan and allow to simmer over medium-low heat until vegetables are cooked through.

Once s uash is done cooking, remove from oven and allow to slightly cool. Turn off oven. Once squash is slightly cooled, scrape the s uash out of the skin and place into medium bowl. Discard skin.

Place cooked s uash in medium bowl and mash with coconut cream. Season with salt and pepper to taste. Place mashed s uash on top of meat and vegetables in the skillet. Serve in the skillet and scoop out portions to put onto plates. Serve warm.

6. Crispy Salmon Arugula Salad

Ingredients

1 wild-caught salmon fillet (about 3 oz.)

1 cup arugula leaves

¼ cup cucumber, diced

2 small radishes, sliced thinly

¼ cup orange segments

¼ cup extra-virgin olive oil, plus 1 tbsp

1 tbsp lemon juice or raw apple cider vinegar

1 tbsp apple cider vinegar Dijon mustard

1 tsp herbes de provence spices (or, a dry Italian spice blend)

Salt and pepper to taste

Instructions

Preheat a large skillet over medium-high heat. Add the 1 tbsp olive oil. Season salmon with salt and pepper, then place in preheated pan and cook the salmon, skin side down for about 3 minutes. Then flip salmon and allow to cook on the other side for about 4 minutes until browned and cooked through.

While salmon is cooking, assemble salad: place the arugula, diced cucumber, sliced radish, and orange segments on a plate.

In a small jar with lid, mix together the remaining olive oil, herbes de provence, lemon juice or apple cider vinegar, and mustard. Shake well to combine.

Place salmon atop salad, and drizzle on dressing to taste.

7. Cinnamon Spiced Orange Slices

Ingredients

2 medium oranges (navel, or caracas are nice varieties)

1 teaspoon cinnamon

Instructions

Peel the oranges and slice them so they make little suns.

Sprinkle with cinnamon. Enjoy!

8. MBA Frittata

Ingredients:

3 eggs

¼ cup chopped fresh asparagus

¼ cup crumbled cooked bacon

¼ cup chopped fresh mushrooms

¼ cup havarti dill cheese shredded 1 teaspoon butter

Directions

Place butter in small skillet or frying pan. Preheat the skillet over medium heat. Beat 3 eggs together and pour it into the skillet. Add crumbled bacon, fresh asparagus, fresh mushrooms and top with havarti dill cheese. Cover with a lid. Frittata is done when the eggs are completely cooked. The frittata will be light and airy and should slide right out of the pan onto a plate. Garnish with fresh fruit. Serve immediately.

9. Muffin Tin Omelet

Ingredients

9 eggs

½ to 1 cup shredded cheese

1 cup chopped or crumbled cooked meat 1 teaspoon dill or other spice

Directions

Turn oven on and pre heat oven to 350 degrees. Place oven rack in center of oven. Beat 9 eggs in a bowl add dill or your favorite spice. Spray muffin tins with cooking spray. Pour egg mixture into muffin tins until ½ full. Add your favorite meat (bacon, sausage, ham or chicken). Add your favorite cheese. You can add your favorite vegetables as well. The muffin tin should be ¾ full.

Bake at 350 degrees for 15 minutes. Insert toothpicks into a couple of muffins, if it comes out clean they are done. Cooking time will vary depending on size of muffin tin and ingredients used. Cool for 5 minutes in muffin tin then remove and serve. Store in refrigerator, microwave for 30 seconds for a   uick easy breakfast.

10. Lox Wrap

Ingredients

Cream cheese

Capers

Diced onion

Lox salmon cured in salt

Pepper

Low carb tortillas

Directions

Spread cream cheese onto low carb tortilla. Add capers, diced onion and pepper. Layer Lox on top of tortilla and roll up like a burrito.

11. Cheeseburger

Ingredients

1 pound ground beef

4 slices of your favorite cheese

3 tablespoons Dale's seasoning

4 low carb tortillas

Favorite condiments for burgers

Directions

In a bowl mix 1 pound ground beef with 3 tablespoons of Dale's seasoning. Shape ground beef into patties. You can make the patties the size you would like. Place oven rack on the top level for broiling burgers. Pre heat broiler use the high setting. Place burgers on broiling pan and broil for 5 to 7 minutes on each side depending on size of burger and how you prefer your burger cooked. Add cheese to burger and return to broiler to melt cheese. Remove from broiler. Wrap in low carb tortilla and add favorite condiments.

12. Taco Salad

Ingredients

1 pound ground beef

1 packet taco seasoning

Shredded cheese

Salsa

Chopped onions

Sliced black olives

Black, pinto or kidney beans

Chopped lettuce

Sour cream

Guacamole or chopped avocados

Chopped tomatoes

Tortilla chips

Directions

Brown ground beef in a pan on the stove. Drain meat using a strainer return to pan. Add taco seasoning packet follow instructions on packet. Place lettuce, onions, beans in a bowl. Add taco seasoned meat top with, tomatoes, avocados, cheese, salsa and black olives. Garnish with tortilla chips.

13. Spaghetti with Spaghetti S uash

Ingredients

1 pound ground beef or mild Italian sausage 2 teaspoons finely diced garlic

1 large can diced tomatoes

2 cans tomato sauce

2 small cans tomato paste

1 teaspoon oregano

1 teaspoon basil

½ cup shredded parmesan, Romano and asiago cheese 1 teaspoon Italian seasoning

1 large or 2 small spaghetti s uash

Directions

Use a cutting board and a large sharp knife cut spaghetti s uash in half. Use a large metal spoon to remove seeds and pulp. Place spaghetti squash in microwave safe bowl, add ½ inch water, cover with plastic wrap and microwave for twenty minutes or until fork tender. Brown ground beef or Italian sausage in pan. Drain meat in strainer. Return to pan and add garlic.

Add diced tomatoes, tomato sauce, and tomato paste. Simmer for 5 minutes. Add basil, oregano and Italian seasoning. Simmer 10 minutes or until thick. Remove s uash from microwave. A fork should go into s uash easily.

Remove the s uash from skin using a large spoon. Place s uash in bowl and separate with a fork. The spaghetti s uash will break up and look like spaghetti noodles. Serve immediately. Place spaghetti s uash in plate add tomato sauce and top with shredded parmesan, Romano and asiago cheese.

14. Chicken Zucchini Alfredo

Ingredients

4 pre cooked chicken breast diced

4 small zucchini s uash sliced julienne

1 bottle Alfredo sauce

½ cup ground parmesan, Romano and asiago cheese Salt and pepper

1 to 2 tablespoons olive oil

Directions

Use a frying pan to sauté zucchini with hot olive oil then sauté for ten minutes until fork tender.

Add Alfredo sauce stir to cover zucchini. Add chicken simmer for 5 minutes until chicken is heated.

Serve immediately. Add ground cheese and salt and pepper for garnish.

15. Butterfinger Shake

Ingredients

2 cups crushed ice

¼ cup heavy cream

¼ cup coconut water

1 tablespoon chocolate protein powder

2 packets Splenda

2 teaspoons peanut butter

Directions

Place all ingredients in a blender. Blend until smooth. Serve in tall glass with a long spoon. Garnish with whipped cream.

16. Chocolate Strawberries

Ingredients

2 cups fresh strawberries

1 cup sugar free chocolate

Directions

Clean strawberries. Set on paper towel to dry, and then place in refrigerator. Melt chocolate in a double boiler until smooth. Remove strawberries from refrigerator and dip each strawberry in chocolate. Place on wax paper to dry then store in refrigerator.

17. Detox Cranberry Lemon Ginger Tea

Ingredients

The juice of 1 lemon

½ cup of cranberries (100 gr)

½ teaspoon of grated ginger root (2 gr)

2 glasses of water (400 ml)

½ teaspoon of cinnamon (2 gr)

½ teaspoon nutmeg (2 gr)

Preparation

First, we will wash the blueberries well and put them in the blender. It is important that all the ingredients are fresh.

We grate the ginger root to get the half teaspoon we need.

We extract the juice of one lemon.

We put the cranberries, the lemon juice, a glass of water and finally the spices in the blender.

We blend until we obtain a homogeneous drink which we then pour into a jug in which we will add the missing glass of water.

The ideal would be to drink a first cup as soon as you wake up and a second one 15 minutes before the main meal of the day

18. Southwestern Steak and Peppers

Ingredients

1/2 tablespoon cumin, ground

1/2 teaspoon coriander, ground

1/2 teaspoon chili powder

1/4 teaspoon salt

3/4 teaspoon pepper, black, coarsely ground

1 pound beef, boneless top sirloin steak trimmed of fat

3 cloves garlic, peeled, 1 halved and 2 minced

3 teaspoons oil, canola divided (or olive oil)

2 medium peppers, red, bell thinly sliced

1 medium onion, white halved lengthwise and thinly sliced

1 teaspoon sugar, brown

1/2 cups coffee, brewed or prepared instant coffee

1/4 cup vinegar, balsamic

4 cups watercress

Instructions

Mix cumin, coriander, chili powder, salt, and 3/4 teaspoon pepper in a small bowl. Rub steak with the cut garlic. Rub the spice mix all over the steak.

Heat 2 teaspoons oil in a large heavy skillet, preferably cast iron, over medium-high heat. Add the steak and cook to desired doneness, 4 to 6 minutes per side for medium-rare. Transfer to a cutting board and let rest.

Add remaining 1 teaspoon oil to the skillet. Add bell peppers and onion; cook, stirring often, until softened, about 4 minutes. Add minced garlic and brown sugar; cook, stirring often, for 1 minute. Add coffee, vinegar, and any accumulated meat juices; cook for 3 minutes to intensify flavor. Season with pepper.

To serve, mound 1 cup watercress on each plate. Top with the sautéed peppers and onion. Slice the steak thinly across the grain and arrange on the vegetables. Pour the sauce from the pan over the steak. Serve immediately.

19. Moroccan Chicken

Ingredients

2 pounds chicken, pieces (breast halves, thighs, and drumsticks) skinned finely shredded

1/2 cup orange juice

1 tablespoon oil, olive

1 tablespoon ginger, fresh

1 teaspoon paprika

1 teaspoon cumin, ground

1/2 teaspoon coriander, ground

1/4 teaspoon pepper, red, crushed

1/8 teaspoon salt

2 teaspoons orange peel

2 tablespoons honey

2 teaspoons orange juice

Instructions

Place chicken in a large resealable plastic bag set in a deep dish. For marinade, in a small bowl, stir together the 1/2 cup orange juice, the olive oil, ginger, paprika, cumin, coriander, crushed red pepper, and salt. Pour marinade over chicken. Seal bag; turn to coat chicken. Marinate in the refrigerator for at least 4 hours or up to 24 hours, turning the bag occasionally. Meanwhile, in a small bowl, stir together orange peel, honey, and the 2 teaspoons orange juice.

Drain the chicken, discarding the marinade. Prepare grill for indirect grilling. Test for medium heat above pan. Place chicken, skinned sides up, on lightly greased grill rack over drip pan. Cover and grill for 50 to 60 minutes or until chicken is done (170°F for breast halves; 180°F for thighs and drumsticks); brush occasionally with honey mixture during the last 10 minutes of grilling.

20. Mini Mushroom and Sausage Quiches

Ingredients

8 ounces sausage, turkey, breakfast, removed from casing and crumbled into small pieces

1 teaspoon oil, olive, extra-virgin

8 ounces mushrooms, sliced

1/4 cup scallions (green onions), sliced

1/4 cup cheese, Swiss, shredded

1 teaspoon pepper, black ground, freshly ground

5 large eggs

3 large egg whites

1 cup milk, lowfat (1%)

Instructions

Position rack in center of oven; preheat to 325°F. Coat a nonstick muffin tin generously with cooking spray (see Tip).

Heat a large nonstick skillet over medium-high heat. Add sausage and cook until golden brown, 6 to 8 minutes. Transfer to a bowl to cool. Add oil to the pan. Add mushrooms and cook, stirring often, until golden brown, 5 to 7 minutes. Transfer mushrooms to the bowl with the sausage. Let cool for 5 minutes. Stir in scallions, cheese, and pepper.

Whisk eggs, egg whites, and milk in a medium bowl. Divide the egg mixture evenly among the prepared muffin cups. Sprinkle a heaping tablespoon of the sausage mixture into each cup.

Bake until the tops are just beginning to brown, 25 minutes. Let cool on a wire rack for 5 minutes. Place a rack on top of the pan, flip it over and turn the uiches out onto the rack. Turn upright and let cool completely.

21. Toasted Steel-Cut Oatmeal With Chai Spices and Caramelized Apples

Ingredients

2 tsp. coconut oil or ghee

1 cup gluten-free steel-cut oats

2 1/2 cups filtered water

1 cup unsweetened coconut, cashew, almond,

or hemp milk

1 tsp. vanilla extract

3/4 tsp. ground cinnamon

1/4 tsp. ground cardamom

1/4 tsp. ground nutmeg

1/4 tsp. sea salt

1/8 tsp. black pepper

2 tbs. coconut oil or ghee

1 tbs. coconut sugar or Sucanat

2 apples, sliced thinly

2 tbs. local honey or pure maple syrup

1/4 cup pecans

Directions

The evening before

Melt 2 teaspoons oil or ghee over medium-low heat in a saucepan. Add oats and toast for two to three minutes, stirring fre uently until lightly golden and fragrant. Reduce heat to low, and carefully pour in the water and milk.

Add vanilla, spices, salt, and pepper, and stir. Remove from heat, cover, and cool; allow to soak in the refrigerator overnight.

In the morning

Melt 2 tablespoons of coconut oil or ghee in a large skillet over medium heat. Add coconut sugar or Sucanat and stir until the sugar begins to melt. Add sliced apples and cook until brown and tender, about 10 minutes.

Meanwhile, return the oats to medium heat and simmer gently, covered, for 15 minutes.

Remove oatmeal from heat, sweeten with honey or maple syrup, top with pecans and caramelized apples, and serve.

Tip: Cinnamon helps regulate blood sugar.

Tip: Healthy fats from pecans slow digestion and balance energy. To make them more digestible, you can soak pecans in water overnight.

22. Asian Forbidden Rice Salad With Mango and Jicama

Salad ingredients

1/2 cup raw cashews

2 cups filtered water

1/2 tsp. sea salt

1 cup black rice

2 fresh mangos, diced

1 small jicama, peeled and diced

1 red bell pepper, diced

1/4 cup chopped fresh cilantro

1/4 cup chopped fresh mint

1 lime, cut into wedges

Dressing ingredients

3 tbs. brown-rice vinegar

1 1/2 tbs. toasted sesame oil

1 1/2 tbs. pure maple syrup

1 tbs. reduced-sodium tamari or coconut aminos

Directions

Preheat oven to 350 degrees F. Spread cashews on a sheet pan and place in the oven until toasted, approximately six to eight minutes. Remove from oven and transfer to a plate to cool.

Combine water, salt, and rice in medium saucepan. Bring to a boil, and then lower heat to low and simmer for 35 to 40 minutes, until all li uid has been absorbed. Fluff the rice with a fork, and then spread it evenly on a parchment-lined sheet pan and allow to cool.

Combine dressing ingredients together in a small bowl. Set aside.

When rice has cooled to the touch, transfer it to a large bowl and combine with mango, jicama, bell pepper, cilantro, and mint. Add dressing to taste and toss until well coated.

Garnish with toasted cashews and serve with lime wedges.

Tip: Whole foods that are deep colored — black, blue, or dark purple — are high in antioxidants and phytonutrients, which reduce inflammation.

23. Moroccan Chickpea and Vegetable Stew

Ingredients

2 tbs. ghee or coconut oil

1 onion, diced

3 cloves garlic, minced

1 tbs. freshly grated gingerroot

2 carrots, chopped

2 celery stalks, chopped

1 1/2 cups chopped cauliflower

4 cups low-sodium vegetable or chicken broth

1 15-oz. can coconut milk

1 to 2 cups filtered water

1 cup dry   uinoa, rinsed

2 to 3 tbs. ras el hanout

1 15-oz. can chickpeas, drained and rinsed

Sea salt and black pepper

3 cups chopped Swiss chard

Toasted coconut (optional)

Fresh cilantro (optional)

Directions

In a large soup pot, heat ghee or oil over medium heat. Sauté onion, garlic, gingerroot, carrots, celery, and cauliflower for five to six minutes.

Add broth, coconut milk, water, uinoa, and ras el hanout, and bring to a simmer. Simmer for 15 minutes to allow uinoa to cook thoroughly.

Add chickpeas and cook for an additional two to three minutes. Season with salt and pepper.

To serve, place about a ½ cup of chopped Swiss chard in the bottom of each soup bowl and cover with soup. Stir well and allow chard to wilt. Garnish with toasted coconut or fresh cilantro, if desired.

Tip: Substitute orange cauliflower, if available, for a boost in carotenoids, a phytonutrient that supports skin and eye health.

24. Grassfed Beef, Red Bean, and Quinoa Chili

Ingredients

1 tbs. ghee or avocado oil

1 medium yellow or white onion, diced

2 cloves garlic, minced

1 lb. lean ground grassfed beef

1 1/2 tsp. sea salt

2 tbs. chili powder

1 tbs. ground cumin

1/2 tsp. ground cinnamon

1 14.5-oz. can diced tomatoes

1 15-oz. can tomato sauce

1/2 cup dry uinoa, rinsed

1 cup filtered water, plus more to thin, if desired

2 15-oz. cans kidney beans with no salt added, drained and rinsed

1 cup frozen organic corn (optional)

Directions

Heat ghee or oil over medium heat in a large heavy pot. Sauté the onion and garlic for three to four minutes, until onion is translucent.

Add the beef, salt, and spices. Using a wooden spoon or spatula, break up beef into smaller pieces and continue to cook an additional three to four minutes, until browned.

Stir in tomatoes, tomato sauce, uinoa, water, beans, and optional corn. Cover and simmer for 15 to 20 minutes. The chili will thicken as it cooks; thin with additional water if desired.

Serve with guacamole or other toppings, if desired.

Tip: The avocados in guacamole are a good source of healthy fats, which can help reduce inflammation and balance hormones.

25. Golden Turmeric Milk

Ingredients

2 cups unsweetened coconut, cashew, almond, or hemp milk

1 tbs. local honey or pure maple syrup

1 tsp. ground turmeric

1 tsp. ground cinnamon

1 tsp. freshly grated gingerroot or 1/4 to 1/2 tsp. ground dried ginger

Dash of black pepper

2 organic chai green tea bags (optional)

Directions

Pour all ingredients except the tea bags into a small saucepan.

Bring to a gentle boil while whisking until spices are well incorporated.

Reduce heat and simmer for five minutes to allow flavors to blend.

Whisk again and serve, or add the chai green tea bags and steep for two to three minutes before serving, if desired.

26. Ras el Hanout Spice Blend

Ingredients

2 tsp. ground cumin

1 tsp. ground coriander

1 tsp. ground ginger

1 tsp. ground turmeric

1 tsp. sea salt

1 tsp. ground cinnamon

3/4 tsp. paprika

3/4 tsp. black pepper

1/2 tsp. cardamom powder

1/2 tsp. ground allspice

1/4 tsp. ground nutmeg

1/4 tsp. ground cloves

1/2 tsp. cayenne pepper (optional)

Directions

Combine spices and stir until well mixed.